The Passenger

Understanding Grief and Loss of a Loved One...

Dr. Paul A. Rodríguez

Cogito Consulting

@2014

Introduction and Purpose

Introduction

Death is a difficult subject for all human beings to face. We are not really supposed to talk about death. For all individuals, the death of a parent or loved one can be a traumatic event. Many individuals face particular difficulties during bereavements. At the same time, for adolescents, they must struggle with developmental responsibilities and the loss of a loved one. Many studies indicate that individuals develop coping skills about grief. However, there is additional evidence that emphasizes that individuals who are unable to overcome their grief are at higher risk for various diverse behavior problems, morbidity, and even suicide.

Purpose

The book provides a comprehensive written guide for educators, counselors, parents, individuals and adolescents for understanding the grief process. Overall all, the information helps all individuals understand the human element of loss and coping with loss of a loved one. The book enhances the present curriculum in the area of conducting group bereavement counseling, helping parents, adults and adolescents cope with the loss of a love one. Parents and school personnel will gain a greater understanding of the grief process. Individuals will strengthen their own personal feelings about death and become well informed about the many aspects of death education. This opportunity will enable individuals to help young people and themselves to understand the reality, to comprehend the inevitability, and to explore the mystery of life and death. Primarily, understanding the developmental stages of how the concept of death unfolds for children enables school counselors and adults to comprehend how children conceive their own grief. The developmental stages strengthen the counselor and adult's competence to utilize counseling strategies for successful grief sessions.

Objectives

The learning objectives include the following:

1. Addresses how children's developmental understanding of death influences the way adolescents and adults grieve.
2. Gives specific knowledge about how children and individuals grieve.

3. Describes techniques and activities that encourage grief peer groups for young people and adults.
4. Give knowledge for understanding why children and individuals hesitate to participate in grief and loss group counseling.

Review of the Literature

The literature survey indicates that few models exist for conducting peer group counseling. A written comprehensive guide for conducting bereavement counseling increases the school counselor's ability to help adolescents and adults during a difficult time in their lives. Likewise, human beings will acquire and develop strengths as they cope with grief.

Many school counselors lack the time and the specialized training needed to conduct extended bereavement counseling with individual teenagers and adults. All individuals benefit from group work; school counselors are in a position to be able to affect the amount and kind of support provided to bereaved teenagers and adults. The reviewed literature indicated that American children encounter loss quite frequently in modern society. Death is a difficult subject for all human beings to face. It becomes crucial and important that educators, school counselors, and parents familiarize themselves with how adolescents and people grieve, and what concerned adults can do to expedite healthy mourning in young people as well as adults.

Synopsis

In conclusion, the long–term goal for conducting bereavement is for the adolescent and all individuals to develop skills and tasks that are necessary for entry into adulthood and life skills for every human being . Individuals will learn to understand the reality, to comprehend the inevitability, and to explore the mystery of life and death. Indubitably, a more profound meaning and goal may emanate when one ponders the subject of death. In so doing, life and death become tangible concepts when the illusion of our earthly immortality is repudiated and when the irreversible inevitability of the death of others and one's self is challenged. The pricelessness of life becomes manifest and obvious when we courageously choose to conscientiously know ourselves, as The Passenger in life.

ACKNOWLEDGEMENT

I dedicate this project to my children Paul Anthony, Alexander Faustino, and Harmonie Mae Rodriguez, may this document serve as a tool and an example for their future endeavors in the pursuit of knowledge, life, and education; and, for my grandchildren, Elijah, Luna, Carson, Maggie, and future generations.

Lastly, for all individuals who have lost loved ones. May this project help them cope with their loss, so that they may be free to live more healthy lives.

Posthumously, for my parents Maria Fernandez Rodriguez (R.I.P. 1991) and Salvador Zuñiga Rodriguez (R.I.P. 1992).

Chapter 1

INTRODUCTION

A counselor's perspective is an important step in developing student and adult support groups. Helping individuals cope with fears and crises can be addressed by using a variety of resources and interventions. The counselor must broaden their perspective on student and individual fears and crises. In so doing, the groundwork for developing specific programs can be addressed.

A client's developmental history determines their response to death and crisis. Current literature suggests that client response to events should be viewed from both an age norm and their understanding and response to death, risk taking, and fears.

Identifying programs and practices can assist counselors in developing programs geared toward crisis prevention or group bereavement counseling. Several programs and practices for helping students and adults cope with fears and crises emphasize a schoolwide orientation and are useful for parents, teachers, and administrators as well as for counselors and adults.

WHAT WE KNOW

Death is a difficult subject for all human beings to face. In adolescents, as well as for adults, the death of a parent or loved can be a traumatic event. Many adolescents face particular difficulties during bereavements. At the same time, they must struggle with developmental responsibilities and the loss of a loved one. Many studies indicate that adolescents develop coping skills about grief. However, there is additional evidence that emphasizes that adolescents who are unable to overcome their grief are at higher risk for various diverse behavior problems, morbidity, and suicide. Sugar (1968) and Van Eerdewegh, Bieri, Parrilla, and Clayton (1982) stated that adolescents are no longer protected by the childhood coping mechanisms of denial, concrete thinking, and immature cognitive skills.

An individual and adolescent's inability to cope with grief may impede the developmental tasks necessary for emotional emergence into adulthood. Beck, Seti, and Tuthill (1963) believed that long-term consequences may include later adult depression. Likewise, Hepworth, Ryder, and Dreyer (1984) indicated that this unresolved depression can lead to rapid courtship combined with a tendency to shun intimacy.

In many cases, the surviving parent may lack the emotional resources to sufficiently help their child. In some cases, the grieving parent may send their child to a psychotherapist that is usually met with resentment and anger. Likewise, the surviving parent may assume that the child will take the deceased parent's role. This in itself complicates and confuses the grieving child. Friends may try to help, but usually have the opposite effect. Moore and Herlihy (1993) reported that friends try to help, but adolescents who have lost a parent report those friends who have not shared the experience do not really understand.

Many school counselors lack the time and the specialized training needed to conduct extended bereavement counseling with individual teenagers. However, because individuals, and adolescents benefit from group work, school counselors are in a position to be able to affect the amount and kind of support provided to bereaved teenagers.

PURPOSE OF THE STUDY

The purpose of this book is to develop a comprehensive written guide for counselors, parents, adults and adolescents to understand the grief process. The literature survey indicates that few models exist for conducting peer group bereavement counseling. Keysiak (1985) described a school-based group for adolescents who had lost a parent or loved one. A written comprehensive guide for conducting bereavement counseling will enhance the school counselor's ability to help adolescents during a difficult time in their lives. Likewise, adolescents, as well as adults, will acquire and develop strengths as they cope with grief. The long-term goal for conducting bereavement counseling is for the adolescent and individual to develop skills and tasks that are necessary for entry into adulthood and life.

Lastly, parents, adults and school personnel will gain a greater understanding of the grief process. Individuals will strengthen their own personal feelings about death and become well informed about the many aspects of death education. This opportunity will enable individuals to help young people to understand the reality, to comprehend the inevitability, and to explore the mystery of life and death.

IMPORTANCE OF THE BOOK

The importance of the book is that school counselors, parents, and adolescents will have an available comprehensively written guide and model for understanding the grief process. Likewise, the guide will readily enable the individual to understand the various aspects about grief bereavement.

The reviewed literature indicated that American children encounter loss quite frequently in modern society. Hayes (1984) estimated that one-third of American children will lose a parent by death before 18 years of age. Fox Valley Hospice (1987) acknowledged that grief is a normal reaction to loss, whether it is a person, place, thing, or idea. Likewise, Jewett (1982) stated that for children, no matter how trivial the loss, the same process must be gone through each time.

It therefore becomes crucial that school counselors and parents familiarize themselves with information about how adolescents grieve, and what concerned adults can do to expedite healthy mourning in young people. In so doing, this guide will assist counselors and adults dealing with adolescents who have experienced loss.

Most importantly, this guide will enable school counselors to be informed about adolescent grief, utilize strategies for successful group peer grief counseling, and realize the importance of parent consultation. All these interventions can mean the difference between adolescents who bear unresolved grief indefinitely, and those who can face the provocation of their grief with support and finally, resolution.

Summary and Considerations

The topic of Death is very difficult to discuss. Many people fear the issue of Death. There are few guides and examples, if any, available for guidance counselors, adults, and educators to follow or review, in understanding the steps and process of grieving. In human society, the ritual of the death of an individual can be very cultural, secular, monetary and/or religious. Other individuals have created Death Cafes to help individuals discuss and deal with the death of a loved one. Death Cafes deal with the human essence and tries to help individuals cope with death through a spiritual and mystical experience. We must be open to discuss the various methods individuals use to cope with the loss of a loved one. While, the secular-thinking individual deals with death as a natural but as nihility, or emptiness. This is odd because the nihility becomes the afterlife. The idea of nothingness becomes the something, yet we cannot comprehend this idea of a one-sided coin.

Educators, adults, and parents become empowered with the death of a student or individual when they understand their own personal feelings and bereavement on the loss of a loved one. We know that everyone deals with death in a special way, and there are no time limitations. However, what I know is that individuals, who are unable to cope with the death of a loved one or loss of a student, and dwell for an extra ordinary time, need professional counseling. Self-reflection and discussion with other individuals helps most individuals cope with loss.

Chapter 2

THE LITERATURE

THE BEGINNING

Past research assumed that children were unable to grieve because it was believed that children had no concept of death, could not comprehend the loss, and would be unable to handle the pain of loss. Freudian theory heavily influenced the concept that grief required sophisticated death concepts.

On the contrary, Nagy (1959) indicated that information collected enables individuals to better understand how a child's concept of death develops over time and that children do grieve in their own way, based on their developmental understanding.

Much of the reviewed literature, that addresses grief in young people, indicates that adults and peers can play a vital role in facilitating grief counseling for young people. The most important adults for children at the time of loss are parents. Also, mental health professionals can facilitate a family in crisis.

McGlaufin (1992) stated "counselors and parents familiarize themselves with how children conceptualize death and loss, how children grieve, and what concerned adults can do to facilitate healthy mourning in children" (p. 11).

The reviewed literature, herein, will:

1. Address children's developmental understanding of death and how this influences the way adolescents grieve.
2. Give specific knowledge about how children grieve.
3. Task of Mourning.
4. Describe techniques and activities that encourage grief peer groups for young people.
5. Give knowledge for understanding why clients hesitate to participate in grief and loss-group counseling.
6. Address the role of the school counselor with bereaved adolescents.

UNDERSTANDING WHAT YOUNG PEOPLE WORRY ABOUT

It is important to understand children's concept of death in order to understand the nature of grief. When school counselors, adults, family members, and school personnel comprehend the fears and concerns of students and individuals, they can appropriately address their needs. In so doing, students and individuals are able to cope with life and enjoy a certain degree of happiness. What young people and adults experience is a great deal of stress and anxiety.

Stress and anxiety are not interchangeable terms. May (1977) enunciated that anxiety is what people feel when stress is placed on them. It is a reaction to stress. Stress is the cognitive component of anxiety that generally brings about lowered levels of performance. Morris, Brown and Halbert (1977) stated that this cognitive element is known as worry. All individuals while growing up encounter personal stress. These stresses include: accidents, illnesses, new sibling, relocations, parental separations and/or divorce, death of a loved one, etc.; likewise, children are affected by life changes that affect society generally, such as: inflation, world conflicts, and the energy crunch. Individuals react to these stresses with either behavioral disorders or psychosomatic reactions. Also, major disorders as asthma and juvenile rheumatoid arthritis may arise.

Fear is an essential and normal developmental part of children's lives. In childhood, fears are momentary in nature and appear at or about the same age for children. Robinson III, Rotter, Fey and Robinson (1992) stated "as children learn to deal with each fear in turn, the fears pass on without great disruption, helping the child to learn adaptive ways for coping with fear" (p. 37). However, for some children this can be a more painful experience than for others because they are not able to cope with the experience.

Schachter (1988) claimed that 10% of the children in the United States would develop a phobia during childhood. Also, there is a larger number of children that do not receive treatment for these phobias than those that do. These children affected by fears are adversely hindered in their functioning effectiveness in schools.

Coddington (1972) compiled the significant life events that affected children. The top 14 include:

Rank	Life Event
1	Death of a parent
2	Divorce of parents
3	Marital separation of parents
4	Jail sentence of parent of 1 year or more
5	Marriage of parent to stepparent
6	Serious illness requiring hospitalization of child
7	Death of brother or sister
8	Acquiring a visible deformity
9	Birth of brother or sister
10	Mother beginning to work
11	Increase of number of arguments between parents
12	Beginning nursery school
13	Addition of third adult to family (i.e., grandparent, etc.)
14	Brother or sister leaving home

DEVELOPMENTAL UNDERSTANDING OF FEARS

One of the most important goals for treatment is not the elimination of the fear, but rather the development of appropriate coping strategies that permit adults and children a sense of control over life events with respect for threatening situations. It is essential that the school counselors and professional counselor understand and develop a sense of the developmental conditions of children's fears. Likewise, strategies must be implemented that help children and individuals learn how to effectively cope with normal developmental fears. Strategies must be developed in order to support those children who have problems dealing with fear.

Croake and Knox (1971), Jersild and Holmes (1935), Kellerman (1981), Maurer (1965), Morris and Kratochwill (1983), and Robinson, Robinson and Whetsell (1988) compiled data on children's most common fears.

Age	Fears
0-6 months	Loss of support, loud noises, sudden movement
7-12 months	Strangers, sudden appearances of large objects, loud noises
1 year	Separation from parent, strangers, injury, toilet
2 years	Large animals, dark room, large objects and machines, loud noises, sudden changes in personal environment
3 years	Dark room, masks, large animals, snakes, separation from parent
4 years	Dark room, noise at night, large animals, snakes, separation from parents
5 years	Wild animals, bodily injury, dark, bad people, separation from parent
6 years	Ghosts, monsters, witches, dark, being alone, thunder and lightning
7 years	Dark, monsters, storms, being lost, kidnapping, being alone
8 years	Dark, people (kidnapper, robber, mugger), guns or weapons, being alone, animals
9 years	Dark, being lost, bad dreams, bodily harm or accident, being alone
10 years	Dark, people, bad dreams, punishment, strangers
11 years	Dark, being alone, bad dreams, being hurt by someone, being sick, tests, grades

Age	Fears
12 years	Dark, punishment (being in trouble, bad grades), being alone, being hurt or taken away, tests, grades
13 years	Crime in general, being hurt or kidnapped, being alone, war in general and nuclear war, bad grades, tests, punishment
14+ years	Failure at school, personal relations, war, tests, sex issues (pregnancy, AIDS), being alone, family concerns

Understanding the fear cycle of children enhances the school counselor's effectiveness and enables them to develop strategies for helping children cope with fear. It is important to understand how children and individuals develop effective ways of coping. Robinson III, Rotter, Fey, and Robinson (1992) proclaimed that "fear is the anticipation of or awareness of exposure to injury, pain or loss. A fear object, then, is any object or conceptualization that the child anticipates might cause injury, pain or loss" (p. 38). The child's perception of vulnerability is associated with the degree of the fear.

The fear cycle indicates that the child apprehend an object in relationship to one's sense of self and one's personal resources. In so doing, the child may experience a sense of power and confidence, realize that they have the resources to deal realistically with the fear or threat, do nothing about the fear and/or take some action. In taking action, the child reexamines the potential fear or threat. The amount of action the child surmounts influences the child's perception of the fear or threat. If the child successfully handles the situation, the less vulnerable they feel. However, the less successful they are, the more vulnerable the child feels.

Those children that are more vulnerable may express more concerns about fear objects and approach new situations with increased consternation. Many children are successful, but some retain nonsensical fears with regards to a specific fear or threat. On the outside, the child may handle comparable situations well, but is unable to transfer coping skills to a certain apprehensive situation.

If the child discerns that they are more powerful than the possible threat or fear, they will respond in one way. Conversely, if, the child perceives that they are less powerful, they will react differently. The child's power consists of: security, self-worth, and control. Robinson III, Rotter, Fey, and Robinsons (1992) proclaimed that security is having a sense of well being and safety based on having allies in facing the world and one's environment. Secondly, self-worth is defined as having a sense of confidence that one is capable and of value. Lastly, control involves having a sense of acting on the environment, of exercising influence over one's life, and the things that happen in life. These three factors empower the child to approach tasks and barriers in life.

Adults who care for and encourage children to make friends will develop a sense of security. In so doing, the child augments the ability to explore their world. Rotter and Robinson (1987) stated that children who feel good about themselves develop the confidence to explore and attempt new strategies to overcome fear. Also, children who are given some autonomy in decision-making learn that they have a certain amount of control over their own lives. They understand that they have strengths and weaknesses, and comprehend that coping with predicaments in life is a natural process of life.

Strategies that the school counselor may employ are decision making, problem-solving skills, increasing successful experiences, interpersonal communication skills training, and assertiveness training. Furthermore, the counselor must include consultation with parents and teachers. Such consultation strategies increase the plausibility of success.

The consultation might emphasize helping the parents and teachers understand the fears of the child and developing strategies for helping children acquire a reasonable sense of control, self-worth, and security. The parent can be provided with helpful points on the role of control, self-worth, and security. Likewise, through parent workshops, the do's and don'ts of parenting with regards to children's fears may be explored. Some of these do's and don'ts may include: don't use fear to secure discipline, don't make fun of children's fears, don't dismiss children's fears as fanciful or imaginary, to name a few.

DEVELOPMENTAL UNDERSTANDING OF DEATH

Gray (1992) stated, "one of the major crises people have to face is the death of a parent" (p. 71). Beck et al. (1963); Birtchnell (1970); Brown, Harris and Copeland (1977); and Dennehy (1966) reported an increased likelihood of psychopathology later in life for individuals who have lost a parent during childhood or adolescence. It is important to consider the developmental theories of Piaget (1920) and Erikson (1959) , and the work of Nagy (1959) to elucidate a child's concept of death. Much of the current literature generally concedes that the concept of death in children develops over time in particular, tangible stages, each with distinguishing discernments.

The developmental theory and research on how children discern death supports the unique understanding of children's conception of death. These distinct stages demonstrate the increasing consciousness children form as they mature. The stages begin from the child's limited comprehension of the conclusiveness and causality of death and proceeds to the more complicated ability to comprehend the actuality of death. Also, as the child matures, a complexity of emotions and numerous philosophical inquiries emanate. It is essential to understand the developmental stages of children. In so doing, one grasps the specific characteristics of their grief. Grief, itself is also developmental in nature.

Generally, birth to age five is recognized as the first conceptual stage in the understanding of death. At this age, there is no cognitive acknowledgment or realistic picture of the permanence of death. McGlauflin (1992) stated, "death is often seen as an altered state of life, and is thought about in a magical way or as a magical place" (p. 12). Commonly, the child may believe the deceased person is living somewhere else, and often worries how the corpse survives in the coffin. Likewise, the child at this age may put blame on themselves and on the circumstances for what had happened. Their own behavior before and after the death may be seen as tangible explanations for what has occurred.

The second stage includes children ages five to ten. Developmentally at this stage, children acquire concrete thinking skills, and strive for a sense of autonomy. Though some magical thinking continues, their new cognitive abilities help them wrestle with the arduous thoughts of finality and causality. While children at this stage want to continue thinking death is reversible, they are beginning to grasp death's permanence. Schell and Loder-McGough (1979) believed that children at this time are extremely vulnerable because, while they are only beginning to understand the concept of death, they can now comprehend the pain of loss.

Within this stage, children begin to wonder more about how death occurs and what happens to the body after death. It is important and vital to their cognitive developmental to provide them with this information. Children at this stage are extremely sensitive to the feelings and thoughts of the adults around them. There is a strong need for children to be accepted and treated normally by their peers.

The final stage includes children from age ten through adolescence. This stage enables the child to comprehensibly understand the reality of death. Children can better think abstractly about themselves and the world. In addition, adolescents can now theorize about life after death with their new cognitive inclinations, and about their personal ideology. Also, within this stage many philosophical inquiries about life and death are now conceivable and recurrent. Children feel the reality of death's permanence, yet, their own idealism of the future makes their own demise and plausibility, but the concept unfathomable.

Foremost, understanding the developmental stages of how the concept of death unfolds for children enables school counselors and adults to comprehend how children conceive their own grief. The developmental stages strengthen the counselor and adult's competence to utilize counseling strategies for successful grief sessions.

HOW CHILDREN GRIEVE

It's important to become familiar with the grieving process, how we come to accept the death, deal with the painful emotions it causes, and recover from our grief. Children do conceptualize death at an early age. They develop a more realistic representation as they mature. Bowlby (1980) recognized that "children do mourn and what is needed is to find a model of mourning that fits children rather than imposing an adult model" (p. 101).

Some unique attributes of the grief of children that discern it from that of adults are taken from the Center of Grieving Children (1987) and include: 1. Children are repetitive in their grief, needed to ask questions and talk about similar issues again and again; 2. They act their feelings out physically; and 3. They always grieve as part of a family, not in isolation. Another important quality for grieving children is that it is cyclical in nature. They process their loss at each developmental level with the improved skills and acquire knowledge each new level brings.

Jewett (1982) identified three phases: early grief, acute grief, and integration of loss and grief. Early grief, the initial phase, is characterized by shock, disbelief, a sense of panic and alarm as the child's vulnerability becomes apparent, and denial, with repeated references to the return of the lost person, object, etc.; this phase is understood as the time children attempt to cope with an overwhelming change in their reality.

Acute grief, after the initial shock has passed, is characterized by a display of strong emotions from anger to despair, and feelings and behaviors suggesting intense searching and yearning. Within this phase, the child may be preoccupied, restless, want to bargain for the return of the lost person or object. They may seem very disorganized. Likewise, this phase may last the longest and is more often the most difficult one for the children and the adults close to them.

The last phase, integration of loss and grief, is characterized as a time when the children recognize and integrate the loss into their lives, and seek meaning in the loss. There is a common sense of acceptance and a sense of relief and strength for having survived the loss.

Generally, the literature suggests an initial period of shock and alarm, followed by a time of confusion and strong emotions, with a resolution of sorts as the loss is integrated and accepted. Also, Jewett (1982) contends that it takes 6 to 12 weeks for the worst pain to diminish, and two years or more for the entire process to unfold. It must be remembered that each child grieves in a unique way within the phase and time frame.

Kubler-Ross (1969) observed a similar pattern of reaction in children in acute crisis in response to loss.

1. Shock and denial.

2. Emergence of intense feelings of grief and anger.

3. Bargaining.

4. Depression and hopelessness.

5. Reduction of intense affect, sometimes accompanied by a sense of resolution and recovery or a sense of detachment and withdrawal from social interaction.

Some common themes for grieving children are: abandonment, blame, and vulnerability. These emotional themes may be seen in many children coping with loss or death.

Abandonment is commonly associated with the death of a parent. Children experience a sense of great anger and bitterness, assuming the leaving was purposeful; worthlessness and shame, assuming the parent did not care; fear of separation from surviving adults and lack of trust; sadness; loneliness, yearning and nostalgic desire.

Blame is another common theme for grieving children. It is an outgrowth of the child's developmental understanding of death. There is a strong need for tangible, concrete explanations and blame is a natural development. Children imagine magical explanations and give power to words, thoughts, and events occurring close to the loss. Center for Grieving Children (1987) stated that children may feel guilty, remorse, and self-blame for things said, action taken or not taken; anger at self, deceased or others; frustration; hatred; and great sadness.

Vulnerability is also a common theme. The child senses a significant change in their view of their world. Their sense of control and security in the world he or she knew is different. Jewett (1982) and Watson (1989) pointed out that children may develop fears of others dying, going to new places, and catastrophes happening. In addition, children may feel intense love for the survivors, panic and helplessness, anxiety, despair, confusion, and disorganization.

It can be understood that children's developmental understanding of death encourages a specific manner of grieving. It is different from adult grief, and is conveyed by a number of emotional themes.

TASKS OF MOURNING

Understanding how death affects people, particularly teens, and the best ways to help them through the stages of mourning is important. Oaks (1996) described four tasks bereavement expert Williams Worden lists as:

1. Accepting the death.
2. Reviewing experiences with the deceased and experiencing the feelings associated with the loss.
3. Refilling all the roles and reassigning all the responsibilities of the deceased.
4. Reinvesting in living without the deceased.

It must be kept in mind that as individuals the experience grief may not proceed in neat stages. The grief experience may include two or more stages of mourning simultaneously. Likewise, the stages may be experienced more than once.

Before closure can commence, the reality of the death must be accepted. It is important that all individuals closely acquainted with the deceased know the facts surrounding the death. Explicit details may be omitted because they may be psychologically traumatizing. For some individuals, the death may take some time. However, for most people attending the funeral and viewing the body helps make the death a reality. In some incidences, the shock of death may be so great that some cannot accept it for weeks or even months after the funeral. Oaks (1996) enunciated that "such denial is a self-provocative devices that's healthy for awhile but indicative that help is needed if denial is prolonged" (p. 2).

Many people cope with the death of someone close to them by repeatedly discussing or asking about details of the death and what led up to it. They are trying to understand how the death might have been avoided. Likewise, individuals seem to be searching for validation that the death actually occurred.

The second task of mourning is reexamining the life experiences with the deceased and coping with the emotional pain of loss. It is common to feel sad over the loss, but anger can also be felt. This anger can be directed toward the doctors who failed to save the life, toward God who seems cruel to take a life or anger toward the deceased for dying and causing them so much pain. Many individuals may feel fear, because death reminds them of their own mortality and that of loved ones. Also, there may be feelings including: relief, that the suffering of terminal illness has ended; resentment that others fail to understand the pain of their loss, for seeming so carefree, and still having their family intact. Also, some may laugh instead of cry, even though there is no joy in their hearts.

The arrays of emotional pain are necessary steps in processing the loss of a loved one. However, many people repress their pains, and this curtails their recovery. The repression of feelings may be due to cultural norms. Expression of strong feelings makes some people feel uncomfortable. Oaks (1996) pointed out that "teens in dysfunctional families are very likely to have been taught to repress their feelings and deny the more painful aspects of reality, including the feelings of loss associated with death" (p. 3).

The third task of mourning necessitates the individual to make adjustments to living without the deceased. All the roles and responsibilities that the deceased held will have to be taken on by someone else. At this time, the individual in crisis may need affirmation that all human beings are unique, including the deceased, and that no one can replace anyone else.

The final task of mourning is to let go of the emotional ties felt for the deceased and engage it in other people or activities. The emotional pain should not hamper us to the point that we are apprehensive to venture into other relationships.

The final task is completed when we put an effort into loving another person or involving ourselves in life again.

If all goes well, the consequence of the mourning process is healing, recovery, and renewed interest in life. However, sometimes the grief process goes awry. All this is referred to as dysfunctional mourning. These include chronic, inhibited, and delayed grief. Oaks (1996) stated that "chronic grief is abnormally long and intense, inhibited grief characterizes the individual who represses the death and emotional pain, and delayed grief is grief that does not occur until weeks or even years after the death occurred" (p. 3).

TECHNIQUES AND ACTIVITIES THAT ENCOURAGES GRIEF GROUP COUNSELING

There is a large number of techniques and activities that the literature suggests to encourage grief work for adolescents and individuals. McGlauflin (1992) pointed out that some studies suggested various writing activities such as journal keeping, writing poems, making books of feelings, or drawing a time line with important dates and events. In addition, the group may spend some time mentioning the euphemisms associated with death. The euphemisms may encourage individuals to use reality-based words in the group. Members within the group are encouraged to fantasize what it would be like to be one of the pupils facing the knowledge of the death or impending death of someone close. Also, members may be encouraged to fantasize what it would be like to face one's own impending death.

Guided recall of grief may be utilized to fantasize or recall the death of a person of great importance to their life. Each member of the group may be motivated to fantasize what it would be like to face the knowledge of the death or impending death of someone who is presently very close. Obituary samples may be read to the group, or members may be encouraged to write their obituary or of someone else in the group. Also, each member can be asked to write a eulogy that portrays their life realistically, that emphasized self. Lastly, members within the group may role play the moments of their death that focus on the when, where, how, who is present, and general attitude of the participants.

However, Oaks (1996) encouraged that the following objectives be included in grief counseling. "the students will:

* become aware that we all experience loss and grief in our lifetime
* have the opportunity to express their feelings over a loss in their lives and share their feelings with others
* by acknowledging and sharing their feelings over a loss, begin to work through their grief
* improve their ability to "listen" to others' feelings associated with loss
* increase their awareness of the variety of feelings we may experience with a loss
* be reassured that feelings of grief are normal
* have an opportunity to say things they needed to say to the deceased, including good-bye
* identify who is included in their personal support systems." (p. 16)

Peer-group grief counseling should be seen as a valuable resource for bereaved pupils. In peer-group counseling, activities should be incorporated to stimulate and challenge investigation into particular aspects of death in ways that allow common group experiences to be discussed freely. The group focus on death can help its members to explore their own ideas and cope more effectively when the issue of death is raised. Likewise, personal strengths and weaknesses may emerge in peer group grief counseling discussion and contribute to deeper communication among the group.

WHY CLIENTS HESITATE TO PARTICIPATE IN GRIEF AND LOSS GROUP COUNSELING

Most current studies that involve grief and loss focus on human death and dying. Individuals go through a grieving cycle that revolves around the individual's strength in coping with the loss of a loved one. However, many people feel grief over the loss of anything of value. Stephenson (1994) stated that a loss could also include part of self. This loss is essential to the overall well-being of the individual. It may be physical or mental capabilities, or the personal role one leads. Bennett and Alvarez (1996-1997) explained that "one example of loss could be the empty nest syndrome in which the mother has somewhat lost the role of being a parent" (p. 51). In whatever situation, the counselor should not discount the loss. It is important that the counselor place value on the individual's loss and encourage the person to continue the grief process.

In the review of literature, there was a significant lack of information in the area of grief counseling due to the cause and value of a loss. The lack of significant information may constrain the individual in the participation of a grief group setting. Counselors should understand and consider the individual's perceived loss important, and deal with it in the same value system they would approach the loss of a person. In so doing, conflict within a group can be avoided. Bennett and Alvarez (1996-1997) suggested that the counselor examine their perceptions of loss value, and use a screening device, such as a written questionnaire, that reveals whether or not the individual should be in a one-on-one session instead of a group setting.

THE ROLE OF SCHOOL COUNSELORS WITH BEREAVED ADOLESCENTS

Counselors cannot offer or give assistance if they do not know about their own personal feelings about loss or death. Counselors need to investigate their own personal ideals of loss or death and be comfortable with all types of deaths. They should also be able to remain calm during a crisis. In so doing, counselors may play significant roles in the recovery of teens from the emotional pain of a death.

GRIEF STRATEGIES

Many studies suggest that counselors include parents as consultants in the grief counseling process.

1. The parent's input may be an effective strategy in grief counseling, in that it is directly related to the many variables that affect an individual's mourning.

2. Open communication between parent and child is essential for healthy grieving. This open communication includes honest and straightforward information, without euphemisms.

3. Parents should be advised to be available and patient with the child.

4. Also, nonverbal communication, such as physical closeness, warmth and love are essential.

5. An environment that encourages free expression of feelings is also stressed. Both parent and child are allowed to express their emotions.

6. It is suggested that parents be both positive and negative about the memories of the deceased.

Lastly, the attendance of a funeral for some can be helpful, but too upsetting for others, and missed by those who were not able to attend. Therefore, the child's unique needs, and desires should be considered when the decision to attend a funeral is made.

In working with teens, counselors should be open-minded. When working with teens, Moore and Herlihy (1993) stated that:

1. Counselors who wish to lead a student grief group need to be comfortable in talking about death and grief. The counselor needs to be open and honest and willing to share his or her own feelings.

2. Humor and laughter are a needed counterpoint to grief and loss in this type of group. Counselors should be aware that a wide range of emotions might exist over the life of the group.

3. It is easy to become emotionally involved with these students. Counselors need to keep in mind that students' grief work is their work and know how and when to let go.

4. Despite a popular belief that a 'magic' year or two exists in which the bulk of grieving takes place, grieving is very much an individual process. In reality, there is no timetable.

5. The school counselor can play a unique and vital role in helping bereaved adolescents. Although, many students resent being taken for therapy, they readily accept an opportunity to join with their peers in the familiar school setting. (p. 59)

Finally, counselors can give students' opportunities to mourn in a healthy way, and facilitate their experiences in the tasks of mourning. In so doing, counselors can be an invaluable resource for adolescents at a difficult time in their lives.

SUMMARY AND CONSIDERATIONS

In summary, the school counselor's objective of helping teens and all human beings cope with the grief process requires that the counselor assist individuals, and teens, directly or indirectly, through work with other individuals, parents, and teachers. They can provide some space to allow bereaved teenagers to deal with painful emotions. Counselors may be in a position to provide this space for some teenagers.

It may be difficult to approach bereaved individuals and teenagers about their personal loss. They may be reluctant to talk about it or feel embarrassed they are now viewed as different and in need of help. Counselors can help students feel less stigmatized. In a counselor and student relationship, it is essential that the normality of mourning be continuously stressed. Many helping professionals are often seen as being able to make everything better or healers. They must realize that it is a process they must go through. It is essential that when dealing with bereaved teens to allow them to feel pain. If they are going to reinvest in life in a healthy way, teens must know that it is both acceptable and normal to feel pain.

In exploring the development or treatment of the grief process in group counseling, an eclectic approach is suggested. The interventions mentioned in this study could mean the difference between teens who carry unresolved grief indefinitely, and those who can face the challenge of their grief with support and finally, resolution.

Indubitably, a more profound meaning and goal may emanate when one ponders the subject of death. In so doing, life and death become tangible concepts when the illusion of our earthly immortality is repudiated and when the irreversible inevitability of the death of others and ourselves is challenged. The pricelessness of life becomes more manifest and obvious when we courageously choose to conscientiously know ourselves.

Consider your own feelings and views of death. Your reflection can openly be communicated with a colleague individually, in a group, or with a close friend. For the most part, it is okay to feel uncomfortable, but the key is to understand yourself. Death is part of life; it is the inevitable and should be discussed and shared. TV and other media use the word "passing or passed" because they feel that this is a 'polite way' to speak about human death, or loss of a loved one. However, it might be a way of ignoring, negating the events and process of human death. Any human death is difficult to accept, but are we not all human beings?

Philosophical Considerations

Normal grief cannot be a disorder because it is 'merely an expectable and culturally sanctioned response to a particular event.' Of course, there is one sense in which grief is not normal: it is (fortunately) not true that most people are presently grieving. However, it is normal both in that it is something that the vast majority of people experience at some time in their lives and (more importantly) in that it is a normal response to loss.

However, grief's normality is really no reason not to regard it as a disorder, since many disorders (e.g., influenza) are similarly normal. This point is well made that grief is simply a natural reaction to a life experience, loss of a loved one. Grief is not pathological in nature, and not a disease. Grief is a human attribute responding to a physical, emotional and conceptual trauma. It is a normal human reaction.

Normal grief seems good because it enables people to overcome loss and form new attachments. Grief is healthy in that failing to grieve would itself be symptomatic of an unhealthy lack of emotional engagement, a general failure to respond emotionally to the world in ways which are valuable. Grief is a consequence of our capacity for attachments to people and objects we may lose. Grief is a necessary concomitant of many things that contribute to a good life, including empathy, family and a sense of human connection and community. It is how we cope and understand the process of human grief that begs the necessity to self reflect and to develop coping strategies to understand the loss. Fore, we are not really supposed to talk about death. Most things may never happen: this one will. Being brave lets no one off the grave. Death is no different moaned at than endured.

Not to be here, not to be anywhere, and soon; nothing more terrible, nothing more true... This is what we fear as human beings—no sight, no sound, no touch or taste or smell, nothing to think with, nothing to love or link with, the anesthetic from which none come around.

I am, right now, Resurrection and Life. The one, who believes in me, even though he or she dies, will live. And, everyone who lives believing in me does not ultimately die at all. Do you believe this? (John 11:25-6, The Message)

Self Reflection

Our son, Alexander was born on October 1, 1992. My wife, Doreen was bed ridden during her entire nine-month pregnancy. My Dad moved in with us in August 1992, diagnosed with terminal liver cancer and asbestos. Early one morning, I noticed that my Dad, Sal was awake. I asked Dad, "Why are you up so early?" My Dad responded, "I may not see the sunrise and midnight will come soon. I am a passenger in my own life." My Dad died on October 22, 1992, I witnessed both the beginning of a life, Alex's birth, and the end of another, my Dad within a few weeks. These human events have stayed with me to this day.

Recently, I was diagnosed with a condition called 'Inclusion Body Myositis' that has no known cure. As the condition progresses, I will be unable to walk, feed myself and become dependent on others for help. My muscles are literally wasting away. Soon, midnight will arrive, and I too will not see the sunrise tomorrow.

I am the passenger within my own life. The hour of departure

has arrived, and we go our ways—I to die,

And, you to live. Which is better, God Only Knows?

From the Apology, Socrates (Plato's dialogue)

Once more into the fray,
Into the last good fight I'll ever know,
Live and Die on this Day,
Live and Die on this Day.
--adapted from Shakespeare--

Chapter 3

GRIEF INTERVENTION GROUPS

A GUIDE ASSISTING EDUCATORS AND TEENS THROUGH THE GRIEF PROCESS FOR SECONDARY SCHOOL COUNSELORS AND NURSES

GRIEF INTERVENTION GROUPS FOR EDUCATORS AND TEENS

OUTLINE

1. Introduction

2. Forming the Group

3. Initial Session: Sharing the Event

4. Second Session: The Stages of Grief

5. Third Session: Events after Death

6. Fourth Session: The Changing Family Structure

7. Fifth Session: Family Rituals and Holidays

8. Sixth Session: Closure

9. Considerations and Conclusion

10. Elisabeth Kubler-Ross: Six Stages Through Which People Must Pass When Confronted with Death, Either Their Own or Another's

11. Worden's Tasks of Grief Resolution/Topics for Group Discussion for Grieving Students

12. Exercises to Be Used in Groups for Students After a Loss/Parkes' Stages of Grief

Suggestions to Counselors When Working With Grieving Students

GRIEF INTERVENTION GROUPS

INTRODUCTION

1. **DEATH: a traumatic event for teens and educators. Grieving teens and educators are often a neglected population.**

2. **TEENAGERS:**

    - **Struggle to accomplish developmental tasks as they emotionally enter into adulthood**
    - **They're also trying to accept the death of the loved one**

3. **SYMPTOMS: When not handled properly, teens develop symptoms that put him or her at risk for any of the following:**

    - **Diverse behavior problems**
    - **Morbidity**
    - **Suicide**
    - **Adult depression**
    - **Accelerated courtship seeking comfort**
    - **A tendency to avoid intimacy**

4. **Parents are in the throws of handling their own grief and loss.**

5. The surviving parents expect the child to assume the deceased parents' role complicating the teen's grief process.

6. Friends and other children do not, or may not, understand the depth or complications of the grief process.

7. Counselors lack time to devote to the student in need of grief intervention or they may lack the proper training to meet student needs for this time.

8. Counseling of this student can be beneficial for the student and rewarding for the counselor when done correctly, in a timely manner, and empathetically.

GRIEF INTERVENTION GROUPS

FORMING THE GROUP

1. Identify students who might benefit from the group experience
   - Send a letter to teachers asking them to help identify students who have experienced death of a family member or friend
   - Seek help from administrators, school nurse, or secretaries or counselors from previous feeder school who might know of students who have had a recent death in their family before entering your site

Interview with each student
   - Use this interview to screen students
   - Determine more about students' situation and readiness for group experience
   - Begin to establish rapport and share information about the group
   - Ground rules are discussed emphasizing confidentiality and diverse emotions that group members may experience
   - A counselor is to emphasize that person's grief is individual and there are no expected time lines, sequences, or reactions in grief intervention
   - Assurance is given that no student will be sent back to class upset and that support from the facilitator and other counselors will be available after group sessions if needed

2. When hesitancy is seen, assurance can be given that the group is open so students can attend once or twice or only when they wish.

3. Define class size. Ideal size of group is 6-8 members.

4. Letters of permission are sent home before the group begins.
    - These letters maintain home-school communication
    - They may also open doors of communication between parent and teenager
    - This letter may provide an opportunity for the family to openly discuss feelings

GRIEF INTERVENTION GROUPS

INITIAL SESSION: SHARING THE EVENT

1.   This session begins with introductions, learning names, and a review of group rules and group goals.

2.   Focus on sharing the event. Each student is asked to share the facts of the death; telling who died, how it happened, and any other details of the events surrounding the death. Questions can serve as an invitation to share. Care should be taken, however, to maintain the confidentiality of the prescreening interview.

3.   Remember that this session is a difficult and emotional one.

4.   Time must be reserved toward the end to achieve closure on the session and to restore emotional homeostasis.

   • Guided imagery or a period of deep breathing and relaxation can be used to close the session
   • If time and circumstances permit, group members can go outside and take a breather

5.   Counselors should leave open time to invite upset members to stay and talk.

6.   Because this is an emotional and draining session, counselors should leave time for self processing and restoration of equilibrium.

GRIEF INTERVENTION GROUPS

SECOND SESSION: THE STAGES OF GRIEF

1. This session begins with a teaching unit, a mini lesson on the work of Kubler-Ross (1969) and other theorists. The counselor emphasizes:

   a. Stages of bereavement do not necessarily progress in an orderly prescribed fashion.
   b. It's equally okay to be anywhere in the process.
   c. Grieving is individual.
   d. The lesson provides shared vocabulary and serves as a tool for discussion.

2. Students are readily able to identify with denial, anger, and depression. In the safety of the group, they can share their anger at the fact that both parents, or a significant other person will not be present at important events in their lives.

3. Feelings are discussed—of depression, how depression dissipates and returns, and how confusing this can be. Students find it comforting to learn that others continue to struggle with sneak attacks of sadness, anger, and depression.

4. As the discussion focuses on the acceptance stage, some students feel they have accepted the death, but others discover that they have more emotions to work through.

5. This session focuses on feelings experienced since the person's death, and extending hope through a recognition that there are common emotions in the grieving process.

6. Students learn that they are not alone in feeling angry or experiencing recurring depression and that sharing helps.

7. To close this session, the counselor can distribute a worksheet such as the Grief Resolution Inventory or a similar instrument. The purpose of this is to help students become aware of their initial feelings, and to realize that they are progressing through the grieving process.

GRIEF INTERVENTION GROUPS

THIRD SESSION: EVENTS AFTER THE DEATH

1. Begin with talking about the original event and expand on it. Funerals are a topic of extended discussion. Humor may surface for the first time at this point. They may want to tell stories or talk about getting the giggles in the middle of the funeral.

2. Counselors must convey the attitude that laughter is healthy and acceptable in this type of group.

3. Talking about the funeral may proceed on a serious note. Many students report that the funeral was a helpful source of comfort and closure. Students vary in their reactions to the person's funeral.

4. Discussion centers on what happened when students returned to school and of the reaction of their peers. Friends frequently do not know what to say is unclear and students in groups are uncomfortable when friends try to ignore the death.

5. The subject of dreams is a rich area for discussion at this time. Some students find dreams comforting. Students relate dreams the person who died has come back to visit and to let them know that they are all right. Nightmares and sad dreams are much less common, but they do occur.

6. It is a powerful experience to have a student who has lost both parents in the group. It may have a strong impact on the group and help them gain a new perspective on their own losses.

GRIEF INTERVENTION GROUPS

FOURTH SESSION: THE CHANGING FAMILY STRUCTURE

1. This session focuses on changes in the family structure. Issues include parental dating, shifting positions in the family, blending families, new responsibilities, and gender issues.

2. Concerns emerge such as increased feelings of responsibility, particularly when the student is the oldest child in the family, and being the only male or female family member left in the household.

3. Parental dating is a major concern. Many students express their trust in their surviving parent to make wise choices about dating and possible remarriage.

4. Other students whose surviving parents have begun dating may relate stories about driving away the parent's boyfriend or girlfriend. They feel uncomfortable or threatened having their parent in relationships. Other students have experienced parental dating and development of new relationships and have come to accept them.

5. Students who were not realistic in their expectations may back off from their original positions after hearing from other students.

6. Usually, students who adjust most easily to the idea of someone new in their parents' lives are those whose parents' death was a result of an illness when there was time to process and emotional support available for the entire family unit.

7.   Students typically fear that once a family returns to a stable place, it will be painful to have that stability disrupted by someone new.

8.   Some fears that surface about parental dating are being afraid to care, afraid to love, afraid to accept someone new or have their parent accept someone new, and afraid of being disloyal to the deceased parent.

GRIEF INTERVENTION GROUPS

FIFTH SESSION: FAMILY RITUALS AND HOLIDAYS

1. The topic of family rituals, such as going to the cemetery, opens this session. Some students are comforted by going to the cemetery and some prefer to go alone. Others have not gone and do not plan to go. Some will go to the cemetery the first time after attending a group where it has been discussed. This opens up a wide gamut of emotions and experiences about the issue of visiting the cemetery.

2. Discussions of family issues also include holidays. Groups help students have the opportunity to work through their concerns and to feel better prepared to face the holiday.

3. These sessions provide opportunities to share concerns for those students facing their first holiday without the deceased parent.

4. Emotions concerning Christmas or Chanukah holidays are much more powerful than those of any other holiday. These holidays extend over a lengthy period of time when our culture expects people to feel joyful and generous, and when students are away from the routine of school for an extended period of time.

5. It is tremendously helpful for students who have not been through a Christmas or Chanukah without the deceased parent to listen to students who have already been through the experience. By listening, they realize that they can get through it too, and that the holidays can still have joys although they miss their mom or dad.

GRIEF INTERVENTION GROUPS

SIXTH SESSION: CLOSURE

1. This session is devoted to summing up and archiving closure.

2. Students are to evaluate the group experience and to make suggestions for improvement. Students may make a suggestion that the group continue but it is healthy for the group to end. Students need to get on with their lives. It is also healthy to rest after weeks of intense emotion.

3. Students can come by the counselor's office to talk occasionally, or can join the group next year.

4. The counselor also establishes continuity by asking the group members to help with the rest of the school year with other students who may be in similar situations. With permission, group members can seek students who face loss and discuss it with them. This helps establish bonds and group members are usually eager to help.

Considerations and Conclusion

1. Counselors leading grief intervention groups need to be comfortable talking about death and grief. The counselor does need to be open and honest and willing to share his or her own feelings.

2. Humor and laughter is a needed counterpoint to grief and loss in this type of group. Counselors should be aware that a wide range of emotions may exist over the life of the group.

3. It is easy to get emotionally involved with these students. They are strong, they've been through a great deal at a young age, and their courage and openness is admirable. Counselors need to keep in mind that students' grief work is their work and know how and when to let go.

4. Despite popular belief that a "magic" year or two exists in which a bulk of grieving takes place, grieving is very much an individual process. In reality, there is no timetable.

5. The school counselor can play a unique and vital role in helping bereaved adolescents. Although many students resent being taken for intervention, they readily accept an opportunity to join with their peers in the familiar school setting.

Elisabeth Kubler-Ross: Six Stages Through Which

People

Must Pass When Confronted with Death, Either Their Own or Another's

Depending on individual needs, a person may stay in one stage for a long period of time, move back and forth from one stage to another, or move through each stage in the order listed below.

DENIAL:	This may be expressed by feeling nothing or insisting there has been no change. It is an important stage and gives people a "time out" to recognize. People in this stage need understanding and time.
ANGER:	Often, after denying a situation, people turn around and react. This reacting can be defined as anger. It can be expressed in nightmares and fears and in disruptive behavior. People in this stage need opportunities to express anger in a positive and healthy way.
BARGAINING:	The purpose of bargaining is to regain a loss. Consequently, a promise is made to do something in order to get something in return.
DEPRESSION:	This sets in when the person realizes that anger and bargaining will not work and one begins to understand that a change may be permanent. This is a stage of grieving for whoever or whatever is lost.

ACCEPTANCE: Acknowledgment of a death — a period of calm after release of emotions, demonstrated by a lifting of sadness and a willingness to keep living.

HOPE: Evidence by a revitalization of energy, a renewed interest in old friends, a development of new friendships, and the return of a sense of humor.

WORDEN'S TASKS OF GRIEF RESOLUTION:

1. To accept the reality of the loss is to come face to face with the reality that the person is dead and that reunion, at least in this life, is impossible.

2. To experience the pain of grief is necessary in order to get the grief work done. Anything that continually allows the person to avoid or suppress this pain can be expected to prolong the course of mourning.

3. To adjust to an environment in which the deceased is missing, involves coming to terms with the unfilled roles played by the deceased.

4. To withdraw emotional energy and reinvest it in another relationship. This involves acknowledging what has been shared and the requirement of love needed. When we continue on our journey, we do so without clinging to the love left behind.

TOPICS FOR GROUP DISCUSSION
FOR GRIEVING STUDENTS

1. Feelings of guilt and anger.

2. Difficulties in relations with the surviving parent and other family members.

3. Memories about and hallucinations about the deceased.

4. School problems.

5. Difficulties relating to peers following loss.

6. Dealing with fears of one's own and other's death.

7. The funeral and other rituals related to loss.

GRIEF INTERVENTION GROUPS

EXERCISES TO BE USED IN GROUPS FOR EDUCATORS AND STUDENTS AFTER A LOSS

1. Having group members write down questions that they might be too embarrassed to raise in the group themselves; then a leader presents the question for discussion.

2. Having group members bring a treasured object related to the deceased to the group.

3. Having group members write a letter to the deceased expressing any thoughts or feelings that were left unexpressed at the time of death.

Source: Gray, R. E. (1988) The role of school counselors with bereaved teenagers: with and without peer support groups. *The School Counselors, 36*, 185-193.

PARKES' STAGES OF GRIEF

1. **PHASE OF NUMBNESS:** During this phase, numbness, shock, and denial serve to block partially or totally, the awareness of loss. Though this is generally accepted as the first reaction, some form of denial permeates further stages.

2. **PHASE OF YEARNING:** During this phase, there is an intense longing for and preoccupation with thoughts of the deceased. In this phase, it is the permanence of the loss rather than fact of loss which is denied.

3. **PHASE OF DISORGANIZATION AND DESPAIR:** During this phase, both the permanence and the fact of loss are accepted. This stage begins generally as the intensity of the yearning begins to diminish and depression, apathy, and aimlessness begin to take over.

4. **PHASE OF REORGANIZATION OF BEHAVIOR:** During this phase, depression, apathy, and aimlessness greatly diminish as a rekindling of interest in the future, the enjoyment of things and others, and a sense of direction is evolving.

Chapter 4

PARENT'S GUIDE FOR ASSISTING TEENS AND EDUCATORS THROUGH THE GRIEVING PROCESS

Introduction

Parenting teenagers may be a challenge to the most knowledgeable and experienced parents. But when death is a reality a child must face, the teen may need much more support and understanding than might be expected. Teens react differently than adults to the grieving process. This handbook is designed to give parents information and resources needed to assist their teen through a period of loss and change.

Definitions

Before going further, we must define some of the terms used in this handbook:

Depression: According to Webster's Dictionary (1995), "Depression is a condition of general emotional dejection and withdrawal; greater sadness and more prolonged than that warranted by an objective reason." The American Academy of Child and Adolescent Psychiatry (2013a) discussing symptoms of grief suggested, "Child and adolescent psychiatrists advise parents to be aware of signs of depression in their youngsters" (p. 1):

- Persistent sadness.
- An inability to enjoy favorite activities.
- Increased activity or irritability.
- Frequent complaints of physical illnesses such as headaches and stomach aches.
- Frequent absences from school or poor performance in school.
- Persistent boredom, low energy, poor concentration; or
- A major change in eating and/or sleeping patterns.

Grief: This is the combination of sorrow, strong emotion, and the resulting confusion which comes from the loss of a family member, friend, or pet. It may feel as though the world is falling apart, that the mourner cannot breathe, is in complete shock and perhaps denial; there is a distinct change in sleeping or eating patterns. Illness may be the end result brought about by emotional strife.

Mourning: Webster's Dictionary (1995) defines mourning as, "a period during which a bereft person grieves." Grief is a very personal issue that varies in length of time and depth depending on the individual. Emerging emotions during the mourning period must be experienced and felt fully in order to come to terms with the grieving process.

Symptomatic Changes Indicating Problems

Teenagers are in a stage of development which identity formulation occurs and he or she is beginning the process of separating from parents. It is at this stage where personal change or loss in their lives can become devastating and lead to depression or suicidal tendencies. Often, in a case of an immediate family member's death, the teen is expected to be a strong force supporting other family members in the mourning process. In actuality, the teen may need as much or more emotional support as others within the family.

According to Alan D. Wolfelt, Ph.D. (1996), "at the same time the bereaved teen is confronted by the death of someone loved, he or she also faces psychological, and academic pressures. While teens may begin to look like 'men' or 'women' they will still need consistent and compassionate support as they do the work of mourning, because physical development does not always equal emotional maturity."

Many teens face the death of important "others" due to auto accidents, shootings, or even suicide. Family dynamic changes such as divorce or separation from a sister or brother through marriage can lead to a sense of loss. Other factors leading to the grieving process might be sexual abuse or molestation, dating, or an abortion. Any of these changes may leave the teens confused, frightened, or even extremely angry and seeking answers. Teenagers may experience shock, have difficulty sleeping or eating or exhibit just the opposite – sleeping all the time or eating too much as in an eating disorder, lacking energy, or have other physical symptoms leaving them unable to function normally.

Each teen may face a unique and complex grieving process. The emotions he or she experiences may be overwhelming and inconsolable leaving the teen feeling depressed and in extreme situations, suicidal. Any long-term denial of these emotions can lead to severe problems later, both psychologically and physiologically.

Teens may react to grief by exhibiting shock or disbelief at the news of the death. Nightmares, disbelief, looking for the deceased person, uncontrollable crying, irritability, or difficulty in communication may be signs of shock. They may react by increasing sexual activity as a means of seeking emotional and physical closeness or indulging in excessive alcohol or drug use as a means of dealing with the pain.

GUILT AND SUICIDAL SYMPTOMS

There may be indications that your child is experiencing problems with the grieving process and is feeling guilty about some aspect of the situation. The American Academy of Child and Adolescent Psychiatry, (2013b) stated, "Younger children . . . believe they are the cause of what happens around them. A young child may believe a parent, grandparent, brother, or sister died because he or she had once 'wished' the person dead. . . The child feels guilty . . . because the wish 'came true" (p. 1) Some danger signals to watch for being:

- An extended period of depression in which the child loses interest in daily activities and events
- Inability to sleep, loss of appetite, prolonged fear of being alone
- Acting much younger for an extended period
- Excessively imitating the dead person
- Repeated statements of wanting to join the dead person
- Withdrawn from friends, or
- Sharp drop in school performance or refusal to attend school"

Guilt is an emotion commonly felt in times of crisis such as death. Falk Funeral Homes, Inc. (1995) indicated in their internet website that, "Whether rational or not, appropriate or not, almost everyone experiences guilt. Guilt can be triggered by almost anything, but usually comes under the heading of "I could have, I should have, I wish I would have . . ." Acknowledge guilt, by looking at each situation, write it down if you need to. If you feel your guilt is warranted, write an apology—even if you are the only one to read it. Vow to learn from your mistakes and move on."

In extreme cases, a teen may turn guilt and emotional problems into a crisis. They may contemplate suicide and must have immediate intervention by a professional who can help. Teens do not realize that the emotions they feel are temporary and there are other venues for handling the pain felt. Professional support must be sought before teens are out of control and attempt suicide. According to the American Association of Suicidology (1997), there are very distinct signs of suicidal tendencies, "These are some of the feelings and things they experience:

- Can't stop the pain.
- Can't think clearly.
- Can't make decisions.
- Can't see any way out.
- Can't sleep, eat or work.
- Can't get out of depression.
- Can't make the sadness go away.
- Can't see a future without pain.

- Can't see themselves as worthwhile.
- Can't get someone's attention.
- Can't seem to get control."

How Can You Help Your Teen and Yourself?

There are some basic tips that can be suggested for helping your teen through this time of crisis. Here is a list of suggestions:

- Talk to your teen. Share your pain with him or her explaining how you feel, what you're doing to handle the pain, and what you expect to happen in the future. Give them a sense that others feel the same pain as they do and can manage it in a positive manner as a means of "healing." This communication shows they're not different from others nor are they alone.
- Listen to the teen as he or she describes their pain, dreams, experiences with death, feelings, etc.
- Acknowledge their pain—don't try to take it away.
- Seek an early diagnosis and medical treatment for depression. Identify professional help such as a Marriage and Family Counselor, school counselor, psychologist, or religious leader.

Address the issue of anger. CyberPsych (1998), an Internet Website, suggests, "What is making you angry with this person? Talk or write out all your feelings about that person or situation. Understanding your anger is the first step toward dealing with it. Hit a pillow, kick a bed, play tennis, or scream if it makes you feel better! The experts claim that exercise is an excellent stress reliever."

- Join a bereavement group.
- Involve the teen in personalizing and planning the funeral. According to Armstrong Funeral Home's (1995) Webpage, "Some ways people personalize the funeral services are:
  - Placing photos and favorite belongings of the deceased in the room.
  - Filling the room with favorite flowers.
  - Substitute traditional organ music with favorite music.
  - Writing a personal letter to the deceased and placing it in the casket.
  - Having children participate in the service.
- Asking people to write a memory about the person who died to be given to family members."
- Don't forget to hug your teen and give him or her support, as they need it.

REFERENCES

American Academy of Child and Adolescent Psychiatry. (2013a). *The depressed child.* Retrieved from http://www.aacap.org/AACAP/Families_and_Youth/Facts_for_Families/Facts_for_families_Pages/The_Depressed_Child_04.aspx

American Academy of Child and Adolescent Psychiatry. (2013b). Facts for families: *Children and grief.* (No. 8). Retrieved from https://www.aacap.org/App_Themes/AACAP/docs/facts_for_families/08_children_and_grief.pdf

Armstrong Funeral Home. (1997). *Talking about death is crucial to the healing process.* Retrieved from http://www.funeral.net/info/ofsa.html

Beck, A. T., Seti, B. B., & Tuthill, R. W. (1963). Childhood bereavement and adult depression. Archives of General Psychiatry, 9, 295-302.

Benett, G. E., & Alvarez, R. K. (1996-1997). Grief and loss: Client resistance in group sessions based on value and cause. California Association for Counseling and Developmental Journal, 17, 51-53.

Birtchnell, J. (1970). Early parent death and psychiatric diagnosis. Social Psychiatry, 7, 202-210.

Bowlby, J. (1980). Attachment and loss (Vol. 3). New York: Basic Books, Inc.

Bowlby, J., & Parkes, C. M. (1970). *The four stages of grief.* Retrieved from http://www.whatsyourgrief.com/bowlby-four-stages-of-grief/

Brown, G. W., Harris, T., & Copeland, T. (1977). Depression and loss. British Journal of Psychiatry, 112, 1049-1069.

Center of Grieving Children. (1987). *The Center for Grieving Children where families find hope and love.* Retrieved from http://www.cgcmaine.org/about-us/

Coddington, D. R. (1972). The significance of life events and etiologic factors in the diseases of children. Journal of Psychosomatic Research, 16, 205-213.

Croake, J., & Knox, F. (1971). A second look at adolescent fears. Adolescence, 6, 279-284.

CyberPsych. (1998). *Cyberpsychology: The intersection of technology and human experience*. Retrieved from http://www.cyberpsychology.com/

Dennehy, C. (1966). Childhood bereavement and psychiatric illness. British Journal of Psychiatry, 112, 1049-1069.

Erikson, E. (1959). *Erik Erikson*. Retrieved from http://www.simplypsychology.org/Erik-Erikson.html

Falk Funeral Home, Inc. (1995). *What is grief?* Retrieved from http://www.grief.com/general.htm

Fox Valley Hospice. (1987). Child grief: A teacher handbook. Bataira, IL: Fox Valley Hospice.

Gray, R. E. (1992). The role of school counselors with bereaved teenagers: With and without peer support groups. (Report No. ISBN-1-56109-040-9). Ann Arbor, MI: Eric Clearinghouse on Counseling and Personnel Services. (Eric Document Reproduction Service No. Ed 340 987).

Hayes, R. C. (1984). Coping with loss: A developmental approach to helping children and youth. Counseling and Human Development, 17, (3), 1-12.

Hepworth, J., Ryder, R. G., & Dreyer, A. S. (1984). The effects of a parental loss on the formation of intimate relationships. Journal of Material and Family Therapy, 10, 73-82.

Jersild, A., & Holmes, F. (1935). A study of children's fears. Journal of Experimental Education, 2, 109-118.

Jewett, C. L. (1982). Helping children cope with separation and loss. Harvard, MA: The Harvard Common Press.

Kellerman, J. (1981). Helping the fearful child. New York, NY: W. W. Norton.

Keysiak, G. J. (1985). Circle of friends. The School Counselor, 33, 47-49.

Kubler-Ross, E. (1969). On death and dying. New York, NY: Macmillan.

Maurer, A. (1965). What children fear. Journal of Genetic Psychology, 10, 265-277.

May, R. (1977). The meaning of anxiety (Rev. ed.). New York, NY: W. W. Norton.

McGlaufin, H. (1992). How children grieve: Implications for counseling. (Report No. ISBN-1-56109-040-9). Ann Arbor, MI: Eric Clearinghouse on Counseling and Personnel Services. (Eric Document Reproduction Service No. Ed 340 987).

Moore, J., & Herlihy, B. (1993/September). Grief groups for students who have had a parent die. The School Counselor, 41, 54-59.

Morris, L. W., Brown, N. R., & Halbert, B. L. (1977). Stress and anxiety (Vol. 4). Washington, DC: Hemisphere Publishing Corporation.

Morris, R. J., & Kratochwill, T. R. (1983). Treating children's fears and phobias: A behavioral approach. New York, NY: Pergamon.

Nagy, M. H. (1959). The child's view of death. In H. Feifel (Ed.). The meaning of death (pp. 79-98). New York, NY: McGraw-Hill Book Co.

Oaks, J. (1996). <u>Death and the adolescent</u>. New York, NY: McGraw-Hill Book Co..

Piaget, J. (1920). Piaget's Theory. Retrieved from http://psych.colorado.edu/~colunga/P4684/piaget.pdf

Robinson, E. H., III, Rotter, J. C., Fey, M. A., & Robinson, S. L. (1992). <u>Children's fears: Toward a preventive model</u>. (Report No. ISBN-1-56109-040-9). Ann Arbor, MI: Eric Clearinghouse on Counseling and Personnel Services. (Eric Document Reproduction Service No. Ed 340 987).

Robinson, E. H., III, Robinson, S., & Whetsell, M. (1988). The study of children's fears. <u>Journal of Humanistic Education and Development, 27</u>, 84-95.

Rotter, J., & Robinson, E. H. (1987). Coping with fear and stress: Classroom interventions. <u>International Quarterly, 5</u>(4), 39-45.

Schachter, R. (1988). <u>When your child is afraid</u>. New York, NY: Simon & Schuster.

Schell, D., & Loder-McGough, C. E. (1979). Children also grieve. In L. Gerber, A. Weiner, A. Kitscher, D. Batten, A. Arkin, & I. Goldberg (Eds.), <u>Perspectives on bereavement</u> (pp. 64-69). New York, NY: Amo Press.

Stephenson, J. S. (1994). Grief and mourning. In R. Bendiksen and R. Fulton (Eds.), <u>Death and identity</u> (3rd ed., pp. 136-176). Philadelphia, PA: Charles Press.

Sugar, M. (1968). Normal adolescent mourning. <u>American Journal of Psychotherapy, 22</u>, 258-269.

Van Eerdwegh, M. M., Bieri, M. D., Parilla, R. H., & Clayton, P. (1982). The bereaved child. <u>British Journal of Psychiatry, 140</u>, 23-29.

Watson, J. (1989/November). Children's concept of death and related feelings. A panel discussion, <u>Children and loss</u>, conducted at Bath-Brunswick Hospice, Brunswick, ME.

Webster's College Dictionary. (1995). New York, NY: Random House Publishers.

Wolfelt, A. D. (1996, summer). *Helping teenagers cope with grief.* Hulse, Playfair, and McGarry Funeral Homes. Retrieved from http://www.hpmc.ca/topic-p.3.htm

www.ingramcontent.com/pod-product-compliance
Lightning Source LLC
Chambersburg PA
CBHW050556280326
41933CB00011B/1864